FLOWING *with* CREATION

Flowing with Creation
100 Birthing Affirmations to Uplift, Nurture, and Support

Written by Rashida A. Marshall
Layout Design by Rashida A. Marshall
Cover Design by Oladimeji Alaka

Copyright © 2024 by Rashida A. Marshall
Published by RAM Enterprises, LLC

All rights reserved. No portion of this book may be reproduced in any form without written permission from the publisher or author; nor may any part of this book be reproduced, stored in a retrieval system, or transmitted in any form or by any means, electronic, mechanical, photocopying, recording, or other, without permision from the publisher,

ISBN: 979-8-218-47276-4
First Edition

*This book is dedicated to the clients and friends from throughout the years who have trusted me to be a part of their pregnancy journey in some way.
Thank you.*

Contents

Introduction..............................11

Breathing Exercise...............13

Affirmations............................15

Meditations & Stretches

Meditation..............................117

Visualization Meditation.....119

Gentle Stretch........................121

Breathing Exercise..............125

Closing......................................127

Introduction

Bringing life into this world is one of the most incredible miracles that we as women possess. As a wellness professional and friend, I have had the blessing to play a role in the pre- and postnatal journey for several clients and friends. Not only have these been amazing learning experiences, but each one has truly reinforced the amount of respect and admiration that I hold for the pregnancy process. The birthing experience is, without a doubt, a unique time for each woman and one that can bring a mix of emotions.

In a society where, often times, little value is placed on us as women, it is absolutely vital that love, care, and encouragement be poured into us as we move through this magical and delicate time in our lives. This is especially important considering the current climate around childbirth often views it as a medical event rather than a natural and miraculous life moment, sometimes increasing feelings of worry and fear. Studies have shown that when a woman is able to approach her birthing experience in a calmer state, it can improve the overall labor experience for both her and baby. To add to this, it may also play a part in enhancing the bonding experience between the mother and her newborn.

It is my utmost belief that every woman who chooses to become a mother deserves to go through her pregnancy with the least amount of stress and the highest level of support. It is for these reasons, among countless others, that I wanted to put together this list of birthing affirmations. And as someone who hopes to one day bring life into this world, these are things that I would want spoken to myself and my baby. As you hear, repeat, and reflect on these words, it is my hope that you continue to build a strong sense of confidence and peace that may support you along your birthing and motherhood journey. Enjoy.

Breathing Exercise

Together, let's move through a calming breathwork exercise to help us with feeling more grounded. If it's currently available to you, take a moment to find a comfortable place to sit or lie down. You may choose to listen to these words during a relaxing walk, bath, or some other activity. Whatever it may be, allow for this moment and space to be dedicated to your self-care.

You may close your eyes or soften your gaze, allowing the eyelids to be heavy. Maybe you choose a sight in the distance on which to focus.

Let your attention center around your breath...feeling the inhale as it enters through your nostrils...and softly parting your lips as you exhale out through the mouth...

Again, deep breath in through the nose, allowing the belly to rise...And exhaling through the mouth, the belly falls...

Take a few more breaths here...calming your mind. If a thought comes about, let it come and go, bringing your attention back to your breathing.

Let's add some length and depth to our breaths. Begin to breathe in on a count of 4-3-2-1...and release 1-2-3-4. Again, slow breath in for 4-3-2-1...and exhale, 1-2-3-4... Together we inhale..4-3-2-1...and exhale 1-2-3-4. Move through one more cycle at your own pace.

Allow your breath to return to a natural inhale and exhale, feeling a sense of calm within your body and mind. As you continue to rest or move at ease, reflect on the following words, either quietly to yourself or repeating them out loud if you would like.

Affirmations

My birthing experience will *flow* just as it should.

I **embrace** the quiet moments when I can connect with my baby.

My body
was
designed
for this.

Each breath I take brings me closer to this *beautiful moment.*

I allow my baby to arrive when he or she is **ready.**

My body is **STRONG.**

My body is **CAPABLE.**

Each moment of my pregnancy journey is **unique**.

I value this *joyous chapter* in my life.

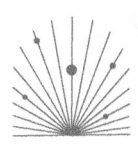

With motherhood will come **new** and **exciting** *joys.*

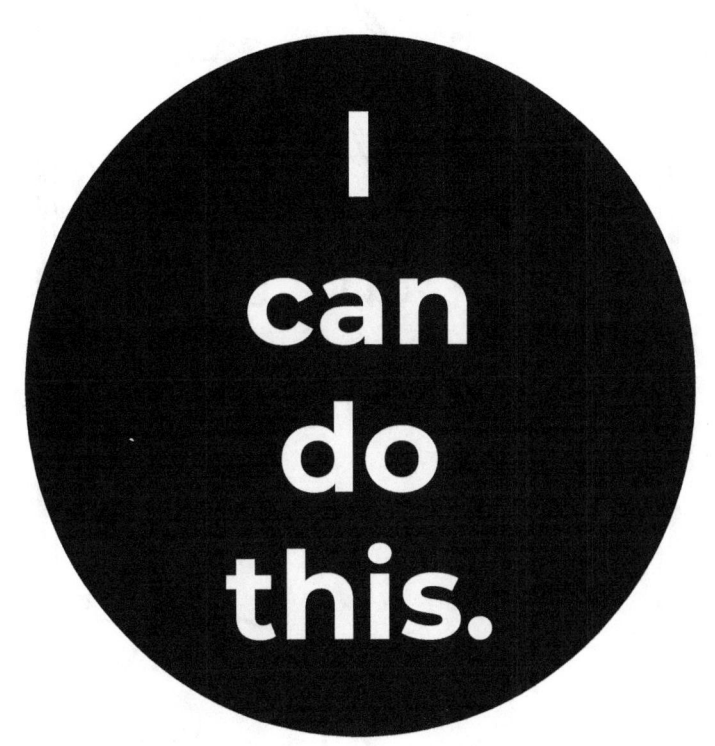

I *honor* my body and all that it does for me and my baby.

I gradually release all tension.

I am
in control
of
my
birthing
experience.

I *release* all self-judgement during this memorable time in my life.

This is **my** *unique* and *beautiful* birthing experience.

I see *beauty* in my pregnancy journey.

Love

&

Gratitude

flow
freely
through
me.

Today, **I choose** to be at **peace** for me and my baby.

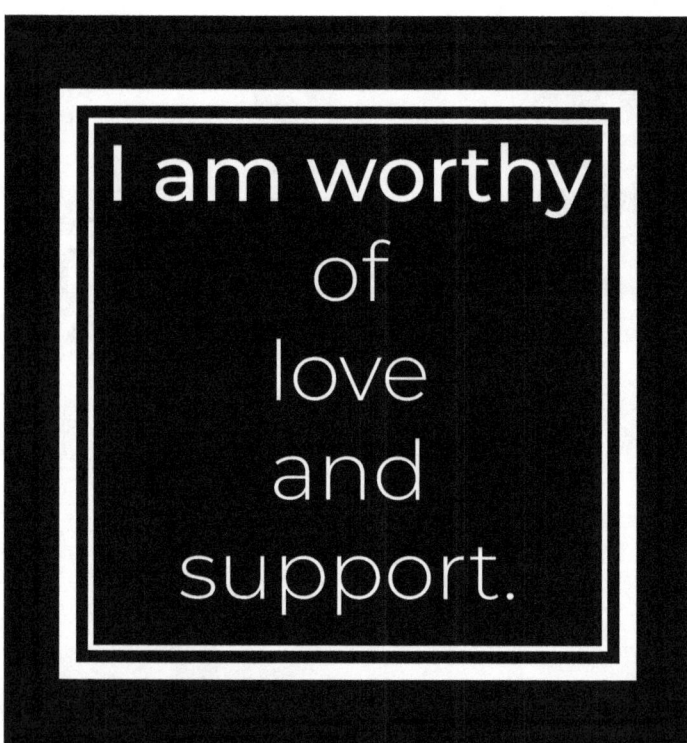

Finding tranquility benefits both me and my baby.

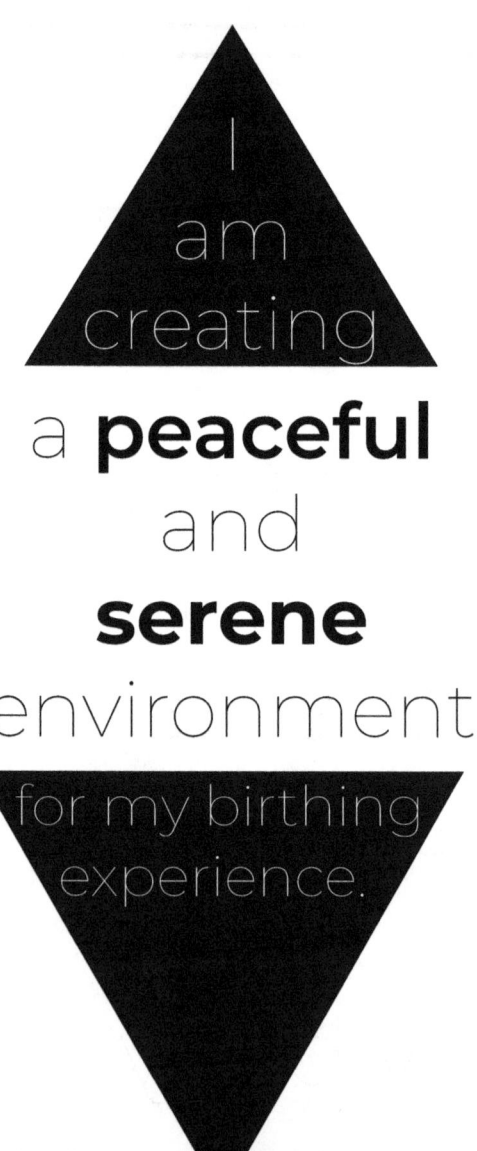

I am creating a **peaceful** and **serene** environment for my birthing experience.

I accept the love and support of those around me.

I am willing to *surrender* to the natural birthing process.

I *cherish* this special moment in my life.

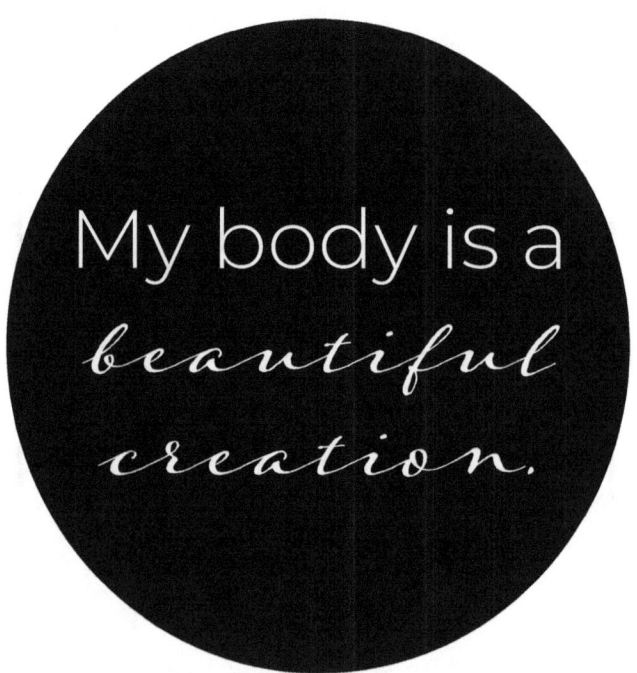

I
believe
and
trust
in my ability
to be a good
mother.

Harmony surrounds me during this special time.

EACH BIRTHING WAVE BRINGS ME **CLOSER** TO MEETING MY BABY.

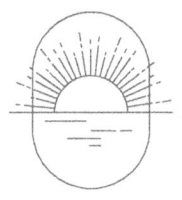

I welcome the release of tension with each breath that I take.

I choose to be generous towards the needs of myself and my baby.

I am willing to bring my baby into a space full of *love, serenity,* and *warmth.*

I speak words of *life* & *love* to myself and my baby.

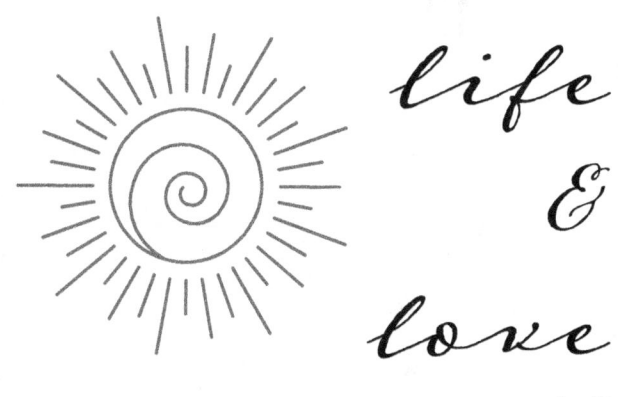

I **open my heart** to this beautiful experience.

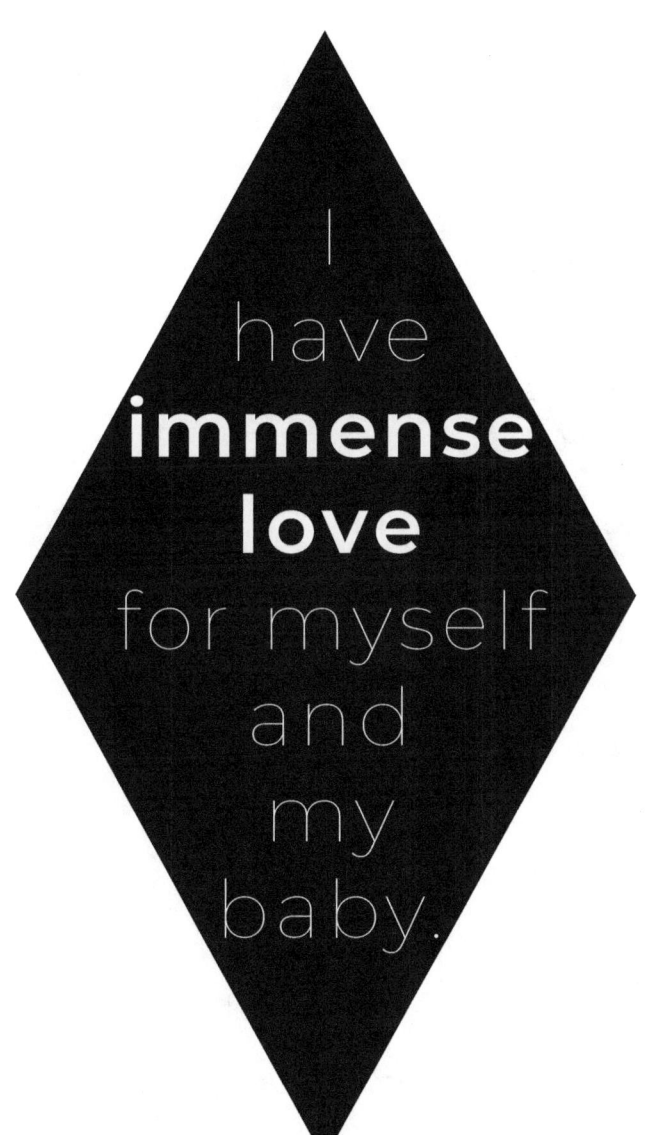

I have **immense love** for myself and my baby.

This *special* time in my life is a *gift* for which I am *grateful.*

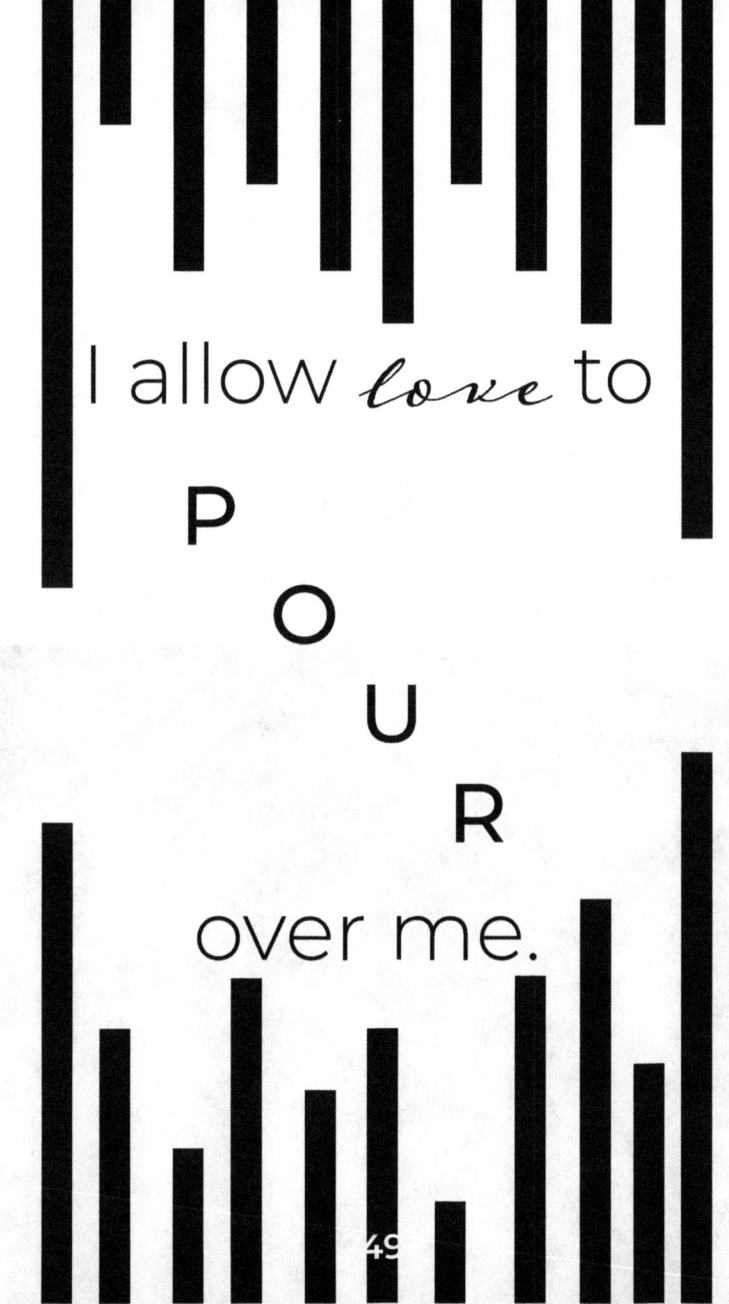

I will cherish the experience of bringing life into this world.

My baby is already surrounded with so much **love** and **joy.**

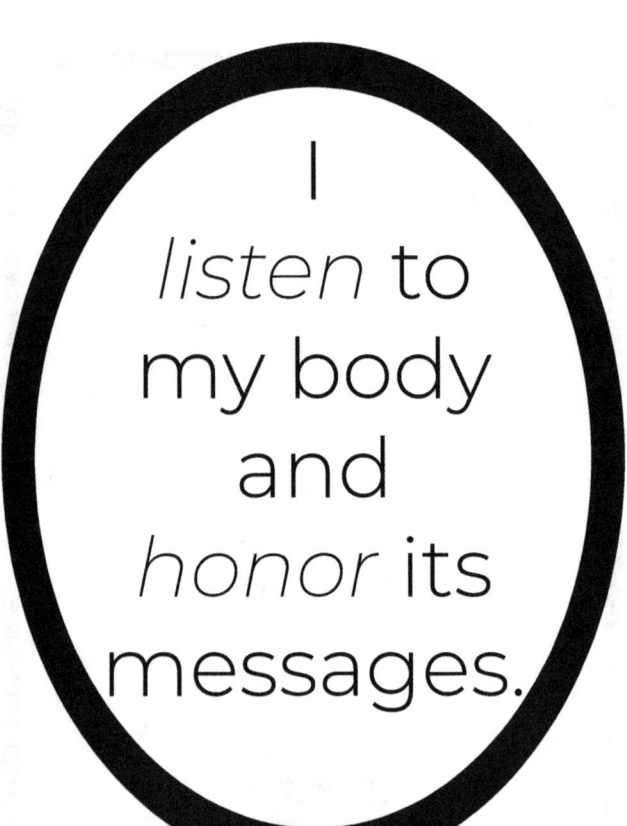

I welcome *this new chapter* in my life.

Each day
I am
learning to
flow
more
deeply
with
my
breath.

I **trust** my body to guide me through this experience.

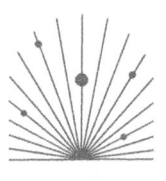

The environment around me is **safe, nurturing,** and **loving.**

I *embrace* my body and all that it is doing for me and my baby.

I allow myself to take a **...pause...** and rest when necessary.

I **RELEASE** ANY JUDGEMENT OR RESENTMENT TOWARDS MYSELF AND MY BODY.

I am filled with joy for the arrival of my baby.

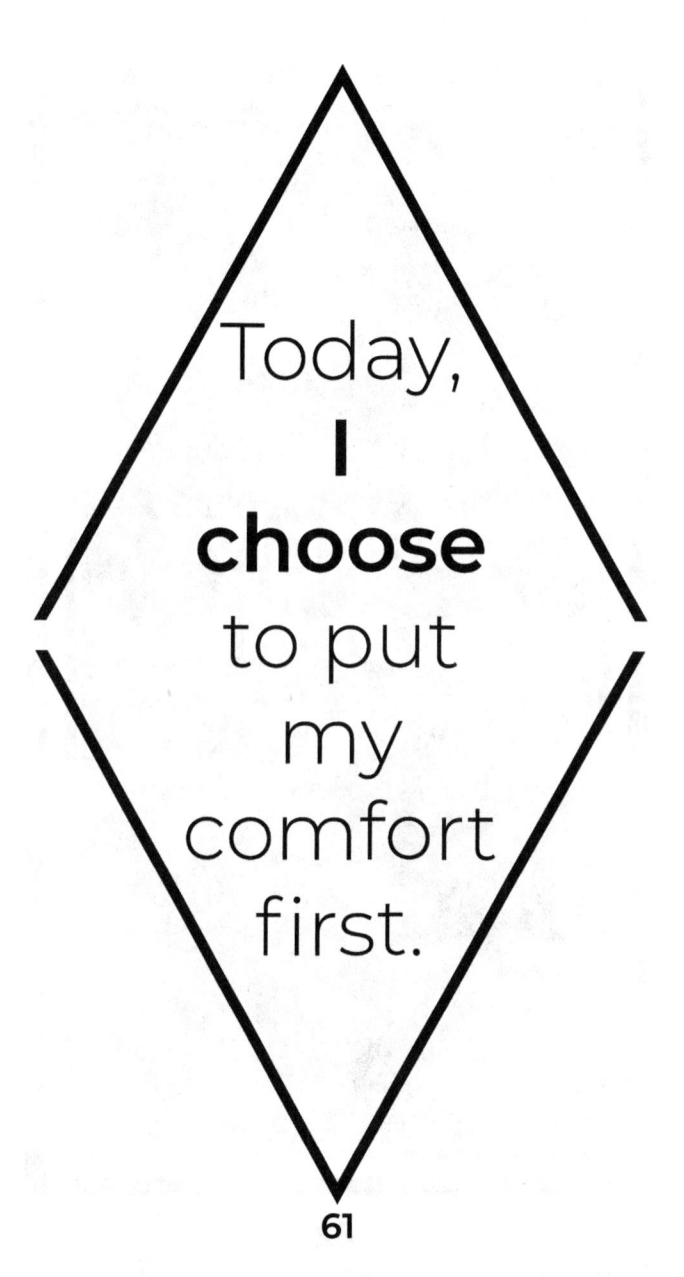

I am **deeply appreciative** of my body.

I allow myself to *evolve* throughout this experience.

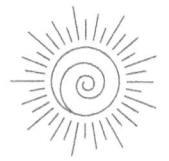

I create
tranquil
and
harmonious
surroundings
for
me
and
my baby.

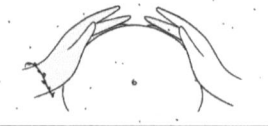

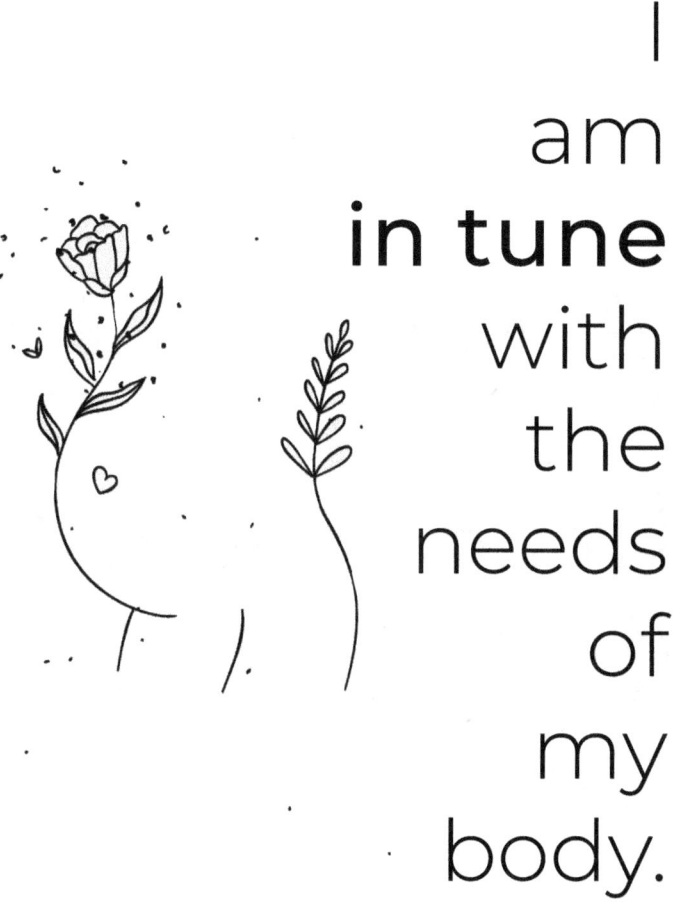

I am **in tune** with the needs of my body.

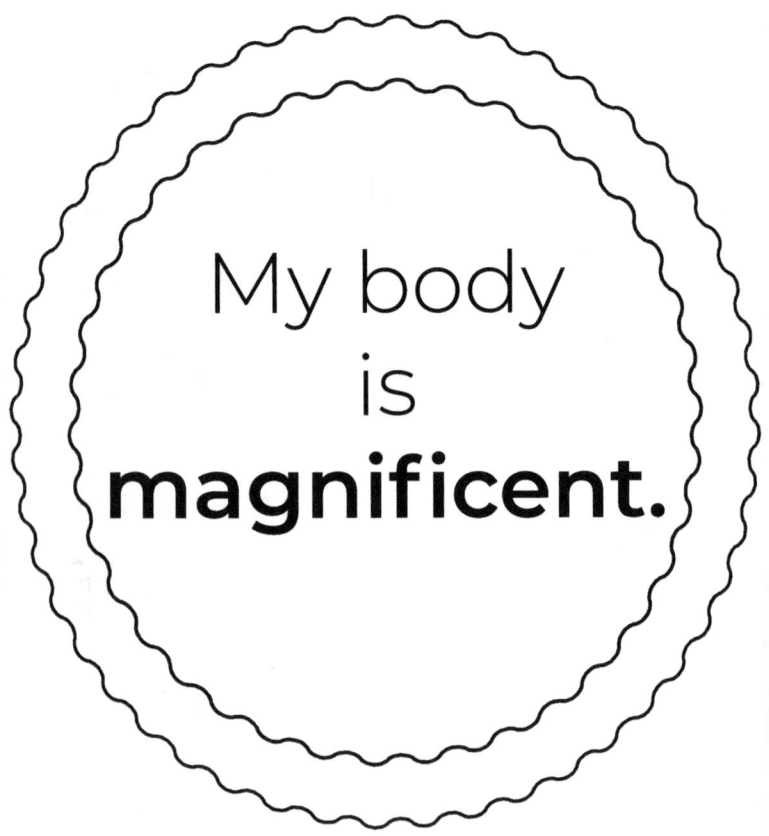

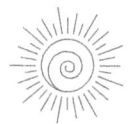

I AM EXCITED
TO BE A PART OF GIVING THE GIFT OF LIFE.

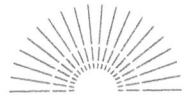

I give thanks
to myself for
creating time
for mental
clarity.

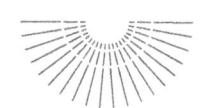

Gratitude and *love* fill my heart.

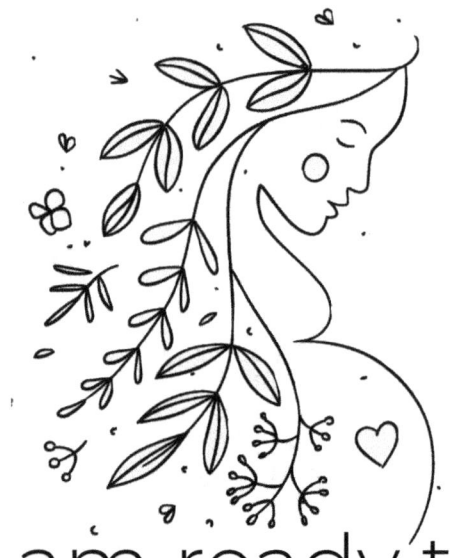

I am ready to step into the role of *motherhood*.

My power lies in my ability to trust the process.

Each breath connects me to a sense of serenity.

I choose to advocate for the well-being of myself and my baby.

My heart **OVERFLOWS** *with joy.*

I deserve to
treat my body
with
love
and
respect.

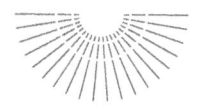

The
thought
of
my baby
fills me
with

happiness.

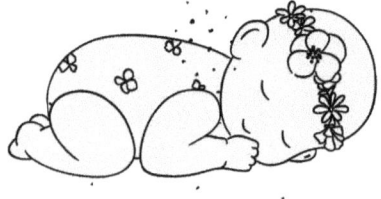

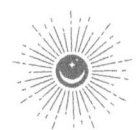

I PRACTICE BEING **INTENTIONAL** ABOUT WHAT I ALLOW TO INFLUENCE MY BIRTHING EXPERIENCE.

I place **no expectations** on myself during this time.

I **WELCOME** THE LESSONS, GIFTS, AND JOYS OF **MOTHERHOOD.**

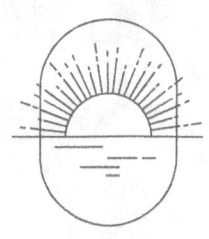

Each day, I learn to **trust the process.**

I am *committed* to the
health
and well-being
of me
and
my baby.

My body is capable of *extraordinary* acts.

I MARVEL AT THE BEAUTY OF CREATION.

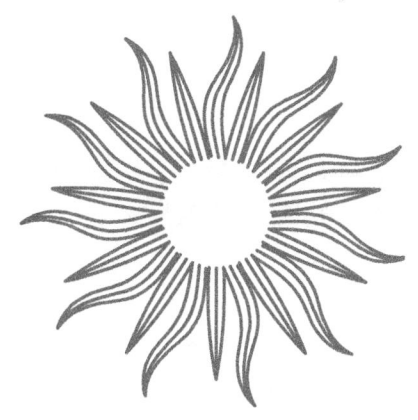

I am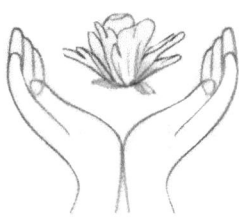
at peace
with each breath that I take.

My baby is a **phenomenal** gift in my life.

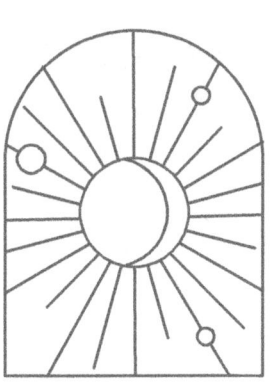

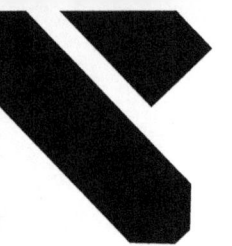

I WELCOME ALL MOMENTS OF SOLITUDE TO **CONNECT WITH** *MYSELF, MY THOUGHTS, AND MY FEELINGS.*

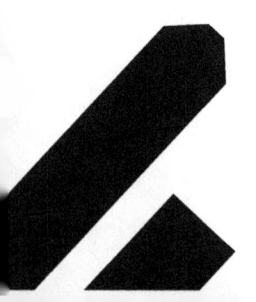

I am **grateful** to be having this experience.

We are surrounded by **love, kindness, and warmth.**

I am in
awe of the
beauty
of life.

I **appreciate** those who support and respect my birthing journey.

I **FREE** MY **HEART** AND **MIND** OF ANY SELF-LIMITING BELIEFS.

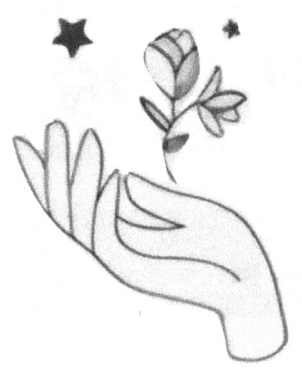

Connecting to my breath and my body puts me at ease.

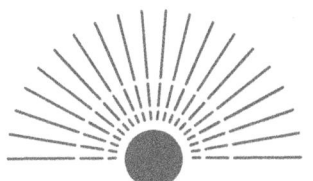

Today is another opportunity to embrace my birthing journey.

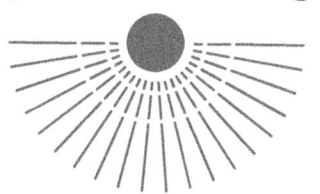

I
AM
AMAZING.

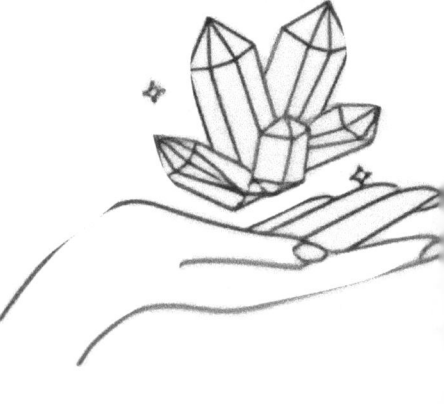

I choose to **put** the needs of **myself** and my baby **first**.

A *serene* energy flows through me.

My birthing experience is SPECIAL *and* WORTHY OF *my acceptance.*

I am grateful for the loving energy that surrounds me.

Each
breath
that I take
nourishes
me
and
my baby.

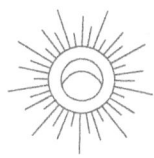

I CHOOSE TO FIND JOY IN THESE SPECIAL MOMENTS.

I give myself *grace* as I move through this new life experience.

I release feelings of fear, worry, and uncertainty.

I am **in awe of all that my body is doing** for both me and my baby.

My feminine energy is **divine**.

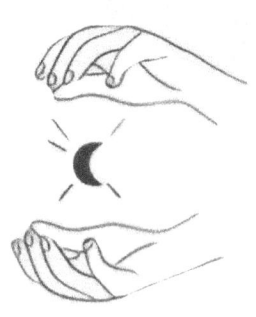

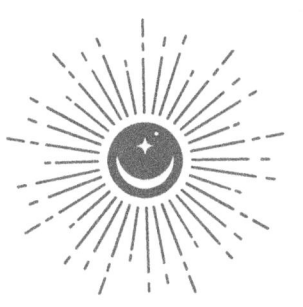

I am
deserving of
happiness
and
bliss.

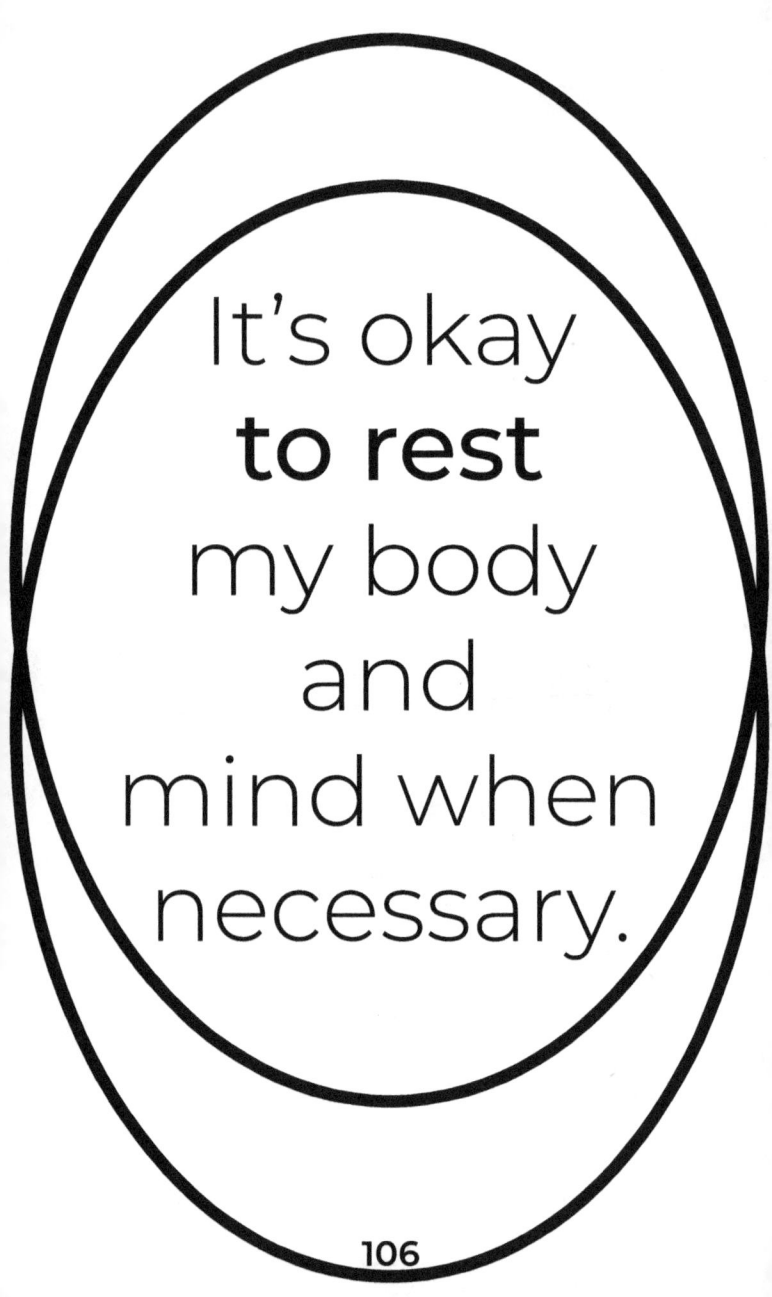

I choose to create time for moments of **self-care** and **self-reflection**.

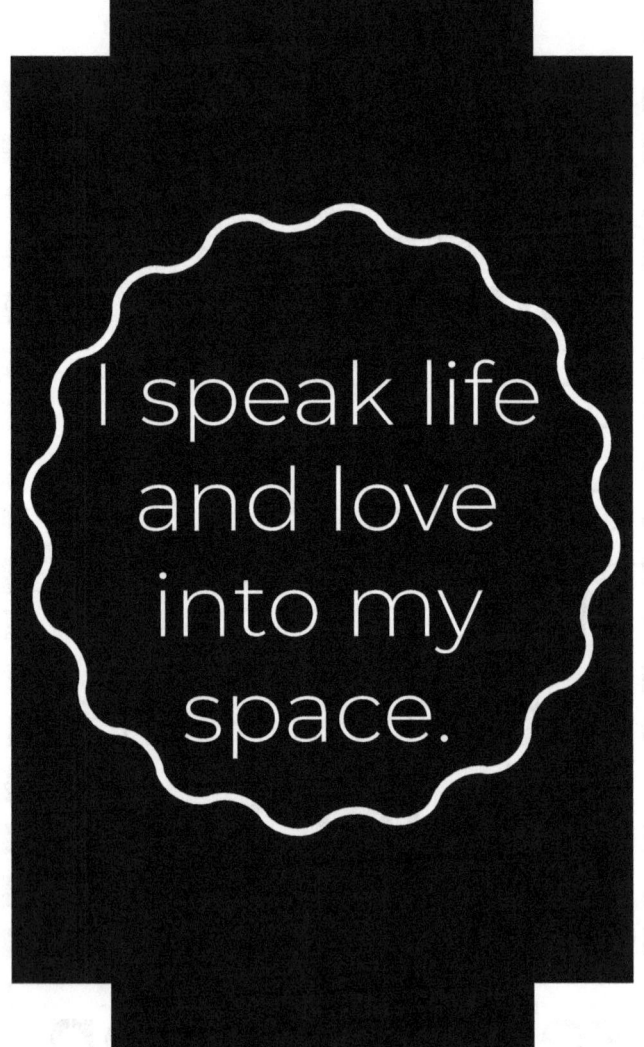

I **value** these moments of *peace.*

I WELCOME THE **EVOLUTION** THAT IS TAKING PLACE IN MY LIFE.

Today, I will be present during each moment of my pregnancy journey.

My baby is a **phenomenal blessing.**

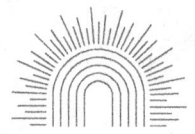

My heart is so full.

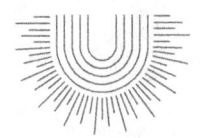

Meditations & Gentle Stretch

Meditation

Welcome to this meditation focused on creating a feeling of being grounded and tranquil.

Let's start by finding ourselves comfortable. You may choose to sit or recline, letting your arms rest comfortably by the sides.

Softly close your eyes or gaze downwards... In this moment, simply breathe...feeling the body become heavy where you sit or lay.

Continue focusing on your breathing... noticing the sound of your inhales and exhales...feeling the belly rise and fall. If any thoughts arise, simply allow them to come and go, like clouds in the sky...returning your attention to your breath. Inhale...exhale. Deep breath in...and out.

Allow the breath to return to a natural, steady flow...and as you breathe reflect on the following statements...

Like water, a sense of tranquility flows through me with each breath...inhale...exhale

In this moment, I am grounded, present, and still...inhale and exhale...

I can always return to my breath for a sense of peace...inhale...exhale...

I breathe in serenity and exhale out uneasiness...inhale and exhale...

I am connected to each moment through the breath...inhale...exhale...

Continue to breathe, allowing these words to sit with you.

Gently begin to bring awareness back to the body...deepening the breath...Maybe wiggling the fingers and toes...or gently rocking from side-to-side...together, let's take in a breath...and release. Once more, breathing in...and exhale...when you're ready, open your eyes...

Thank you for taking the time out to enjoy this mediation.

Visualization

Welcome to this visualization exercise where we will bring to mind an image of a calm, serene environment.

Take a moment to find yourself in a comfortable place, maybe seated or reclined. Allow the arms to rest comfortably, either by your sides or on your lap. Softly close your eyes or gaze downwards to the ground.

Begin to bring attention to your breathing. Inhale through your nose...exhale out through the mouth. Breathing in and out. Feel the belly rise with each inhale...and fall with each exhale.

See yourself in a beautiful, scenic park...all around you is soft, green grass. Breathtaking flowers. Out in the distance are magnificently lush trees. The sky is a crisp, light blue. The rays of the sun shine down against your face.

Start to imagine the gentle breeze that whisks across your skin...feel the light, cool air...notice the leaves on the trees as they flow softly, swaying in the wind...hear the sounds of the breeze...

Picture yourself comfortably relaxed in this space. Maybe you're laying back in the grass looking up at the sky. Perhaps you're seated on a bench gazing out into the distance.

What else is a part of this scenic, peaceful environment? Butterflies fluttering near the flowers? A serene lake in the distance? Birds singing in the sky? The sounds of water in a nearby fountain?

Continue flowing with your breath as you feel yourself in this space.

Take in a deep breath through the nose and

exhale. Again, deep breath in and release. When you're ready, open your eyes. Thank you for joining me. Return to this visualization exercise as often as needed.

Gentle Stretch

Find yourself in a comfortable seated or standing position. Allow your body to feel heavy and firmly rooted in your space. Your arms rest comfortably by your sides. Start with taking in a deep breath...and exhale.

Take another breath, and as you exhale allow your head to tilt to the right, bringing the ear closer to the shoulder. Feeling the stretch along the left side. Inhale and lift the head to center, exhale as it tilts to the left, releasing tension along the right.

The inhale breath lifts the head into center, and as you breathe out, lower the head and bring chin to chest. Now, flow with your breath as you flow through a neck rotation. The head moves over to the right, now back as you look up to the ceiling, over the left and back in center, chin to chest. Now reverse – over to the left, up, back to your right and back to center, chin to chest.

Allow the head to lift. Breathe in as you draw the shoulders up, take them around and back, then lower and exhale. Again, for two, inhale the shoulders up to the ears, draw them around and down the back and into center. Reverse the movement, taking it through the two rotations with a steady breath

On your next breath, sweep your left arm out to the side and lift it overhead and over to the right, stretching the side body. Exhale as the arm gently lowers. We switch, lifting the right arm up and over while breathing in, and release as the arm melts back by the side. Again, with the left arm. Inhale and stretch, lengthening through the fingers, and exhale, release. Over to your right, stretch to the high diagonal as you breathe in and exhale lower.

Take in a breath, and as you exhale, bring your chin to chest and begin to round forward and down towards the ground with a soft bend in the knees. Go to whatever distance feels comfortable and available to you during this movement. Inhale as you round back up to standing, stacking the spine in center. The head is the last thing to lift. Again, release the breath as you round down, letting the arms and head be heavy. Inhale as you round back up to an upright position.

Begin to round down again on your next exhale, and now place your hands on each leg, right above the knees. Take a breath in as tilt your head and tailbone to the sky, opening the front of the body. And exhale, bringing chin to chest and rounding the lower back. Again, inhale and look up, drawing the shoulder blades together. Now exhale, rounding the spine and tucking the tail. Move through one more as you continue to connect with your breath.

When you're ready, allow the arms to hang heavy in space as you use an inhale to round back up. Sweep both the hands out to the sides and place the palms behind the back of the head. Breathe in and allow the head to fall back into the hands, as you open up the chest, letting the elbows go back slightly. Exhale as you draw the head back into center. Once more - inhale. The head tilts back as the elbows go wide. And release, coming back upright.

Remove the hands from behind the head as they fall back down by the sides. Turn the palms so they face back. Take a breath in as the palms press back, while looking up toward the ceiling. Exhale, as the arms return to the sides and the head looks straight out in front. Again, deep breath in as the arms sweep back, feeling taller and more lifted. Exhale release.

Thank you for flowing through this gentle stretch session. Revisit as often as needed.

Breathing Exercise 2

As we bring this listening experience to a close, let's take some time to re-center our heart, mind, and body.

Place one hand comfortably on your belly and the other on your heart. Take a moment to return your focus to your breath, closing your eyes if it's available to you. Breathe in deeply, feeling the air pass through the nostrils...and exhale, connecting to a greater sense of peace. Again, draw in a breath...and release.

Allow yourself to take time with each breath in...and out...quieting your mind....hear your inhale and exhale.

Take in one more breath, feeling a deep sense of love and gratitude...and exhale, letting go of any tension or fear within the body...

Deep breath down into the belly, connecting to a sense of peace in this moment...and breathe out, releasing what no longer serves you...

Breathing in, experiencing a moment of appreciation for your body, your mind, your entire being....and exhale...

Continue flowing with your breath....

When you feel ready, gently open your eyes.

Thank you for taking the time out for this breathing exercise.

Closing

Thank you for taking the time out to fill your heart, mind, and spirit with these affirming statements, meditations, and exercises. I encourage you to return to these words as often as you may need to during your pregnancy journey. Until next time, sending you love and light.

www.ingramcontent.com/pod-product-compliance
Lightning Source LLC
Chambersburg PA
CBHW072026060426
42449CB00035B/2705